COMPLETE GUIDE TO LUMBAR DISCECTOMY

Essential Handbook To Expert Insights On Minimally Invasive Surgery, Spinal Disc Treatment, Pain Management, And Recovery Strategies

DR. BRUNO HORAN

Copyright © 2023 by Dr. Bruno Horan

All rights reserved. Except for brief quotations embodied in critical reviews and certain other noncommercial uses permitted by copyright law, no part of this publication may be reproduced, distributed, or transmitted in any form or by any means, Including photocopying, recording, or other electronic or mechanical methods, without the prior written permission of the publisher.

Disclaimer:

The information provided in this book, is intended for general informational purposes only and should not be considered as professional advice.

The author has made every effort to ensure the accuracy of the information presented. However, readers are advised to consult with a qualified healthcare professional before attempting any herbal remedies or making significant changes to their wellness routine. Individual health conditions vary, and what may be suitable for one person may not be appropriate for another.

It is important to note that the author is not in any endorsement deal, partnership, or affiliation with any organization, brand, or company mentioned in this book. Any references to specific products or services are based on the author's personal experience or general knowledge and do not imply an endorsement or promotion of those products or services

Contents

CHAPTER ONE 19
  ANATOMY AND PHYSIOLOGY OF THE LUMBAR SPINE 19
    Detailed Structure Of The Lumbar Spine 19
    Function And Role Of Intervertebral Discs 20
    Nerve Pathways And Their Significance 21
    Common Lumbar Spine Conditions 22
    Impact Of Disc Herniation On The Body 23

CHAPTER TWO 25
  DIAGNOSIS AND EVALUATIONS 25
    Initial Consultation And Physical Examination 25
    Imaging Techniques (MRI, CT Scans) 26
    Differential Diagnosis 27
    Importance Of Accurate Diagnosis 28
    Preparing For Surgical Consultation 28

CHAPTER THREE 31
  SURGICAL TECHNIQUES AND APPROACHES 31
    Description Of Open Discectomy 31
    Microdiscectomy Procedure 32
    Endoscopic Discectomy Details 32

Laser Discectomy Explained 33
Choosing The Right Surgical Approach 34
CHAPTER FOUR 35
PREOPERATIVE PREPARATIONS 35
Necessary Medical Evaluations 35
Preoperative Instructions And Guidelines 36
Lifestyle Changes And Preparations 37
Mental And Emotional Readiness 37
Importance Of Preoperative Fitness 38
CHAPTER FIVE 39
THE SURGICAL PROCEDURE 39
Step-By-Step Description Of The Surgery 41
Anesthesia And Pain Management 42
Duration And Expectations 42
The Surgical Team For A Lumbar Discectomy Typically Includes: 43
Immediate Post-surgical Care 44
CHAPTER SIX 47
POSTOPERATIVE RECOVERY 47
Hospital Stay And Initial Recovery Period 47
Pain Management And Medications 48

Physical Therapy And Rehabilitation 49

Activities To Avoid During Recovery 50

Signs Of Complications And When To Seek Help . 52

Fever Or Chills: A Sign Of Possible Infection 52

CHAPTER SEVEN 55

  LONG-TERM CARE AND OUTCOMES 55

    Long-Term Physical Therapy 56

    Maintaining Spine Health 57

    Lifestyle Adjustments For Better Outcomes 59

    Potential Long-Term Complications 60

    Success Rates And Patient Stories 62

CHAPTER EIGHT 65

  COMMON CONCERNS AND FAQS 65

    Addressing Common Patient Concerns 65

    Detailed FAQ Section 66

    Tips For A Smooth Recovery 68

    Managing Expectations Post-Surgery 70

    Resources For Further Information And Support . 71

ABOUT THIS BOOK

Lumbar discectomy stands as a pivotal surgical intervention designed to alleviate the debilitating symptoms associated with herniated discs in the lower spine. This book, Lumbar Discectomy, delves deeply into the procedure, offering a comprehensive guide that blends medical expertise with practical advice. It begins with a thorough overview, detailing the definition, history, and common causes that necessitate a discectomy, along with the symptoms that indicate its need. Understanding the benefits and high success rates of this surgery sets a hopeful tone for patients and their families.

The intricate anatomy and physiology of the lumbar spine are meticulously covered, offering readers a detailed understanding of the lumbar spine's structure and the critical role intervertebral discs play. The book elucidates the complex nerve pathways and highlights how conditions like disc herniation impact the body.

This foundational knowledge is essential for comprehending the significance of accurate diagnosis and the various imaging techniques, such as MRI and CT scans, used to confirm the condition.

Diagnosis and evaluations are crucial steps in the treatment process, and this book outlines what to expect during initial consultations and physical examinations. The importance of accurate diagnosis is emphasized, ensuring that readers are well-prepared for surgical consultations. The different surgical techniques and approaches are described in detail, from traditional open discectomy to advanced procedures like microdiscectomy, endoscopic discectomy, and laser discectomy. This section helps patients understand the options available and the criteria for choosing the right surgical approach.

Preoperative preparations are covered extensively, providing necessary medical evaluations, preoperative instructions, and guidelines for lifestyle changes. The book emphasizes the importance of mental and emotional readiness and preoperative fitness, crucial for a successful surgical outcome. The surgical procedure itself is explained step-by-step, detailing anesthesia, pain management, and the roles of the surgical team, giving readers a clear expectation of what the surgery entails.

Postoperative recovery is a significant focus, with detailed information on hospital stay, pain management, and physical therapy. The book offers practical advice on activities to avoid during recovery and identifies signs of complications, emphasizing when to seek help. Long-term care and outcomes are discussed to help patients maintain spine health and make necessary lifestyle adjustments for optimal recovery. Success rates and patient stories provide real-life insights into life after surgery.

Addressing common concerns and FAQs, the book ensures that all potential patient questions are covered. It provides tips for a smooth recovery, and managing post-surgery expectations, and offers resources for further information and support. This comprehensive guide is an indispensable resource for anyone considering or recovering from lumbar discectomy, combining medical precision with empathetic guidance.

Overview of Lumbar Discectomy

A lumbar discectomy is a surgical procedure designed to alleviate pain and other symptoms caused by a herniated disc in the lower spine. This condition occurs when the soft, gel-like center of a spinal disc pushes out through a tear in its outer layer, pressing on nearby nerves. The procedure involves removing the portion of the disc that is compressing the nerve, thereby relieving the pain, numbness, and weakness that can radiate from the lower back down into the legs.

Detailed Definition and History

Lumbar discectomy is a minimally invasive surgery performed to excise the herniated part of an intervertebral disc. The goal is to decompress the affected spinal nerve roots and alleviate pain. Historically, the procedure has evolved significantly since its inception. The first recorded discectomy was performed in the 1930s by Dr. Mixter and Dr. Barr, marking a revolutionary step in neurosurgery. Over the decades, advancements in medical technology and surgical techniques have made the procedure less invasive and more effective. Modern lumbar discectomy often utilizes microsurgical or endoscopic techniques, allowing for smaller incisions, reduced recovery time, and lower risk of complications.

Common Causes for Needing Discectomy

Several factors can lead to a herniated disc, necessitating a lumbar discectomy. Age-related wear and tear is the most common cause, as discs naturally degenerate over time, losing hydration and elasticity. This degeneration can make them more prone to tearing or rupturing with minimal strain. Acute trauma, such as lifting heavy objects improperly, sudden impacts, or severe falls, can also cause disc herniation. Genetic predisposition plays a role, with some individuals having a higher likelihood of developing disc problems. Additionally, lifestyle factors like obesity, smoking, and a sedentary lifestyle can contribute to disc degeneration and herniation.

Symptoms Indicating a Lumbar Discectomy

Symptoms that might indicate the need for a lumbar discectomy include persistent lower back pain, often radiating to the buttocks, legs, and feet, known as sciatica. This pain can be sharp, burning, or throbbing and is typically exacerbated by activities like sitting, coughing, or sneezing. Numbness, tingling, or weakness in the legs and feet are also common symptoms, indicating nerve compression. In severe cases, patients may experience a loss of bladder or bowel control, known as cauda equina syndrome, which requires immediate medical attention. When conservative treatments like physical therapy, medications, or epidural steroid injections fail to provide relief, a lumbar discectomy may be recommended.

Benefits and Success Rates

The benefits of lumbar discectomy are substantial, particularly for those who have not found relief through non-surgical methods. Patients typically experience significant pain relief, improved mobility, and enhanced quality of life. The success rate for lumbar discectomy is high, with studies indicating that approximately 90% of patients experience substantial relief from their symptoms. This procedure allows many individuals to return to their normal activities and work with minimal discomfort. The recovery period is generally short, with many patients resuming light activities within a few weeks and full activities within a few months. Advances in surgical techniques have also reduced the risk of complications, making lumbar discectomy a safe and effective option for many patients.

Overview of Non-Surgical Alternatives

Before considering surgery, non-surgical alternatives are often explored. Physical therapy is a cornerstone of conservative treatment, focusing on exercises that strengthen the back and core muscles, improve flexibility, and reduce pain. Medications, such as nonsteroidal anti-inflammatory drugs (NSAIDs), muscle relaxants, and oral steroids, can help manage pain and inflammation. Epidural steroid injections, where corticosteroids are injected into the space around the spinal nerves, can provide temporary pain relief and reduce inflammation. Chiropractic care and acupuncture are other alternative treatments that some patients find beneficial. Lifestyle modifications, such as weight management, smoking cessation, and ergonomic adjustments, can also alleviate symptoms and prevent further disc degeneration. These non-surgical approaches are often successful in managing symptoms and improving quality of life, although they may not provide permanent relief for all patients.

CHAPTER ONE

ANATOMY AND PHYSIOLOGY OF THE LUMBAR SPINE

Detailed Structure Of The Lumbar Spine

The lumbar spine, located in the lower back, consists of five vertebrae labeled L1 through L5. These vertebrae are the largest and strongest in the spinal column, designed to bear much of the body's weight and provide flexibility and movement.

Each vertebra is separated by an intervertebral disc, which acts as a cushion and shock absorber. The vertebrae are connected by facet joints that enable a range of movements such as bending, twisting, and stretching.

The vertebral body, the thick anterior portion of each vertebra, supports the majority of the body's weight. The vertebral arch, located at the back, forms the spinal canal, which houses and protects the spinal cord.

Protruding from the vertebral arch are the spinous and transverse processes, which serve as attachment points for muscles and ligaments. This complex structure of bones, discs, joints, and processes allows the lumbar spine to provide both stability and flexibility.

Function And Role Of Intervertebral Discs

Intervertebral discs are essential components of the lumbar spine, providing both structural integrity and flexibility. Each disc consists of two main parts: the annulus fibrosus and the nucleus pulposus. The annulus fibrosus is the tough, outer layer made of concentric rings of collagen fibers, which provide strength and support. The nucleus pulposus is the soft, gel-like center that acts as a cushion, absorbing shocks and distributing pressure evenly across the disc.

These discs allow the spine to bend and twist while maintaining its stability. They act as shock absorbers during activities such as walking, running, and lifting, preventing damage to the vertebrae and other spinal structures. Additionally, intervertebral discs help to maintain proper spacing between the vertebrae, which is crucial for the normal functioning of the nerve pathways that pass through the spinal column.

Nerve Pathways And Their Significance

The lumbar spine is a critical hub for the body's nervous system. Nerve roots exit the spinal cord through openings between the vertebrae, called foramina, and extend to various parts of the body. The lumbar nerve roots, including the sciatic nerve, are particularly important as they innervate the lower extremities, controlling muscle movements and sensation in the legs and feet.

Any disruption or compression of these nerve pathways can lead to significant symptoms. For instance, nerve root compression can result in pain, numbness, tingling, and weakness in the lower back, buttocks, legs, and feet. Understanding the layout and function of these nerve pathways is essential for diagnosing and treating conditions affecting the lumbar spine, such as disc herniation and spinal stenosis.

Common Lumbar Spine Conditions

The lumbar spine is prone to a variety of conditions due to its role in supporting much of the body's weight and facilitating movement. Some of the most common conditions include lumbar disc herniation, spinal stenosis, spondylolisthesis, and degenerative disc disease.

Lumbar disc herniation occurs when the nucleus pulposus protrudes through a tear in the annulus fibrosus, often compressing nearby nerves and causing pain. Spinal stenosis involves the narrowing of the spinal canal, which can compress the spinal cord and nerves, leading to symptoms like pain, numbness, and weakness. Spondylolisthesis is the displacement of one vertebra over another, which can cause instability and nerve compression. Degenerative disc disease is a condition where the intervertebral discs lose their cushioning ability over time, resulting in pain and reduced mobility.

Impact Of Disc Herniation On The Body

Disc herniation in the lumbar spine can have widespread effects on the body, primarily due to the compression of nerve roots. When a disc herniates, it can press on the sciatic nerve, causing sciatica—a condition characterized by sharp, shooting pain that radiates from the lower back down to the legs and feet. This pain is often accompanied by numbness, tingling, and muscle weakness.

The location and severity of the herniation determine the specific symptoms and their intensity. In severe cases, disc herniation can lead to loss of bowel and bladder control, requiring immediate medical attention. Chronic pain and mobility issues can significantly impact a person's quality of life, making it difficult to perform daily activities and reducing overall physical function.

Understanding the anatomy and physiology of the lumbar spine, along with the implications of common conditions like disc herniation, is crucial for both prevention and treatment. Effective management strategies, including physical therapy, medications, and potentially surgical interventions, can help alleviate symptoms and improve function, allowing individuals to maintain a more active and pain-free lifestyle.

CHAPTER TWO

DIAGNOSIS AND EVALUATIONS

Diagnosing lumbar disc herniation typically begins with an initial consultation and physical examination. During the consultation, the healthcare provider will inquire about the patient's medical history, including any previous back injuries or related symptoms. This information helps to establish a baseline understanding of the patient's condition and potential risk factors for disc herniation. A thorough physical examination follows, focusing on the spine's range of motion, reflexes, and sensation in the legs and feet.

Initial Consultation And Physical Examination

The initial consultation for lumbar disc herniation involves a detailed discussion between the patient and the healthcare provider. The physician will ask about the nature of the pain, its onset, duration, and any activities that exacerbate or alleviate symptoms. Understanding these details helps in formulating a preliminary diagnosis and determining the appropriate course of action.

Following the consultation, a physical examination is conducted to assess the patient's musculoskeletal health and neurological function. This examination typically includes tests to evaluate reflexes, muscle strength, and sensation in the lower extremities. These tests help to pinpoint the location and severity of nerve compression caused by the herniated disc.

Imaging Techniques (MRI, CT Scans)

Imaging plays a crucial role in diagnosing lumbar disc herniation. Magnetic Resonance Imaging (MRI) and Computed Tomography (CT) scans are commonly used to visualize the spine's structures and detect abnormalities such as herniated discs.

MRI is particularly effective in providing detailed images of soft tissues, including the spinal discs and nerves. It helps in identifying the size and location of the herniated disc, as well as any associated nerve compression. CT scans, on the other hand, offer detailed cross-sectional images of the spine and can be used to assess bone structures and detect spinal stenosis or other bony abnormalities that may contribute to symptoms.

Differential Diagnosis

In diagnosing lumbar disc herniation, it's essential to consider other conditions that may present with similar symptoms. Differential diagnosis involves distinguishing between conditions such as spinal stenosis, sciatica, and muscle strain, which can also cause lower back pain and radiating leg pain.

Thorough clinical evaluation combined with imaging studies helps to rule out other potential causes and confirm lumbar disc herniation as the primary diagnosis. This ensures that the treatment plan addresses the specific underlying cause of the patient's symptoms.

Importance Of Accurate Diagnosis

Accurate diagnosis of lumbar disc herniation is crucial for developing an effective treatment strategy. Misdiagnosis or delayed diagnosis can lead to inappropriate treatment and prolonged discomfort for the patient. By pinpointing the exact location and severity of the herniated disc, healthcare providers can tailor treatment options to relieve symptoms and restore spinal function effectively.

Preparing For Surgical Consultation

Preparing for a surgical consultation involves several important steps to ensure that both the patient and healthcare provider are well-prepared for discussion and decision-making. Patients should gather all relevant medical records, including imaging results and previous treatment histories, to provide a comprehensive overview of their condition.

It's essential to prepare a list of questions and concerns to discuss with the surgeon during the consultation. This helps in clarifying treatment options, understanding potential risks and benefits of surgery, and addressing any specific preferences or expectations regarding the surgical procedure and recovery process.

CHAPTER THREE

SURGICAL TECHNIQUES AND APPROACHES

Description Of Open Discectomy

Open discectomy is a traditional surgical approach used to treat lumbar disc herniation that involves making a relatively larger incision in the back.

During this procedure, the surgeon removes the herniated portion of the disc that is pressing on the nerve root or spinal cord.

This technique provides direct access to the affected disc, allowing for thorough removal of herniated material and any fragments that may be causing compression.

It is typically performed under general anesthesia to ensure patient comfort and safety.

Microdiscectomy Procedure

Microdiscectomy is a minimally invasive surgical procedure aimed at relieving pressure on spinal nerves caused by a herniated disc. Unlike open discectomy, microdiscectomy involves making a smaller incision, usually less than an inch long. Through this small incision, the surgeon uses specialized instruments and a microscope to carefully remove the herniated disc material. This approach minimizes damage to surrounding tissues, reduces recovery time, and often allows for same-day discharge from the hospital.

Endoscopic Discectomy Details

Endoscopic discectomy is a modern minimally invasive technique used to treat lumbar disc herniation. It involves inserting a thin, flexible tube with a camera (endoscope) through a small incision in the back. The endoscope allows the surgeon to visualize the herniated disc and surrounding structures on a monitor. Using tiny instruments inserted through the endoscope, the surgeon can remove the herniated disc material and relieve pressure on the spinal nerves. This approach offers advantages such as smaller incisions, less tissue trauma, quicker recovery, and reduced risk of complications compared to traditional open surgery.

Laser Discectomy Explained

Laser discectomy is a minimally invasive procedure used in some cases of lumbar disc herniation. It involves using a laser to vaporize or shrink the herniated disc material. During the procedure, a small incision is made in the back, and a laser fiber is inserted through a thin tube into the affected disc space. The laser energy is then used to target and remove the herniated tissue, decompressing the nerve root or spinal cord. Laser discectomy is often chosen for its potential to minimize tissue damage, reduce recovery time, and alleviate pain associated with disc herniation.

Choosing The Right Surgical Approach

Selecting the appropriate surgical approach for lumbar discectomy depends on various factors, including the location and severity of the herniated disc, the patient's overall health, and the surgeon's expertise. Open discectomy remains a reliable option for cases where direct visualization and extensive decompression are necessary. Microdiscectomy and endoscopic discectomy are preferred for their minimally invasive nature, offering quicker recovery and less post-operative discomfort. Laser discectomy may be considered in specific cases where its advantages, such as reduced tissue trauma and faster recovery, align with patient needs and surgical goals. Consulting with a spine specialist will help determine the most suitable approach tailored to individual circumstances.

CHAPTER FOUR

PREOPERATIVE PREPARATIONS

Before undergoing lumbar discectomy, thorough preoperative preparations are essential to ensure a successful surgical outcome. These preparations typically begin with a series of necessary medical evaluations. Your healthcare team will conduct a comprehensive assessment of your overall health, focusing on your spine condition, medical history, and any underlying health issues. This evaluation may include physical examinations, imaging tests such as MRI scans or X-rays, and possibly blood tests to ensure that you are in optimal health for surgery.

Necessary Medical Evaluations

The medical evaluations for lumbar discectomy are critical in determining your suitability for surgery and identifying any potential risks or complications. Your healthcare provider will carefully review your medical history, including any previous spinal surgeries, existing medications, and allergies. Imaging tests, such as MRI scans or CT scans, will be used to precisely locate the herniated disc and assess its impact on nearby nerves.

These evaluations provide your surgical team with a clear understanding of your spinal condition, allowing them to tailor the surgical approach to meet your specific needs.

Preoperative Instructions And Guidelines

Following the medical evaluations, you will receive detailed preoperative instructions and guidelines from your healthcare team. These instructions are designed to prepare you physically and mentally for the surgery.

They may include guidelines on fasting before surgery, which medications to take or avoid in the days leading up to the procedure, and specific instructions regarding hygiene and skin preparation.

Lifestyle Changes And Preparations

In preparation for lumbar discectomy, adopting certain lifestyle changes can significantly contribute to a smoother recovery and improved surgical outcomes. Your healthcare team may advise you to quit smoking, if applicable, as smoking can impair healing and increase the risk of complications. Engaging in regular physical activity and maintaining a healthy diet can also enhance your overall health and readiness for surgery.

Mental And Emotional Readiness

Preparing mentally and emotionally for lumbar discectomy is equally important. The prospect of surgery can evoke various emotions such as anxiety or fear. It's essential to discuss any concerns or anxieties with your healthcare team and loved ones. Engaging in relaxation techniques, such as deep breathing exercises or meditation, can help alleviate stress and promote a positive mindset before surgery.

Importance Of Preoperative Fitness

Achieving optimal preoperative fitness plays a crucial role in enhancing surgical outcomes and facilitating a faster recovery. By following your healthcare team's recommendations for physical activity and nutrition, you can strengthen your body and improve its ability to withstand the stress of surgery. Maintaining good physical fitness also reduces the risk of complications during and after lumbar discectomy, contributing to a successful surgical outcome.

CHAPTER FIVE
THE SURGICAL PROCEDURE

Lumbar discectomy is a surgical procedure aimed at relieving pressure on the spinal nerves caused by a herniated disc in the lower back.

It's typically performed under general anesthesia to ensure the patient remains unconscious and pain-free throughout the operation.

Surgeons begin by making a small incision in the lower back, directly over the affected disc. This incision allows them to access the spine without disturbing surrounding muscles more than necessary, minimizing trauma and speeding up recovery.

Once the surgical site is accessed, the surgeon carefully moves aside muscles and tissues to reach the spine.

Using specialized surgical instruments and guided by imaging technology like fluoroscopy, they locate the herniated disc that is pressing against the spinal nerve roots.

The next step involves removing the herniated portion of the disc, which may involve trimming or excising the affected area to relieve pressure on the nerves and restore normal spinal function.

Following the removal of the herniated disc material, the surgeon ensures that no fragments remain that could potentially continue to irritate the nerves.

 This meticulous approach aims to optimize the patient's recovery and minimize the risk of future complications.

Once satisfied with the procedure, the surgeon closes the incision using sutures or surgical staples, and a sterile bandage is applied to protect the wound.

Step-By-Step Description Of The Surgery

Incision and Access: The surgeon begins by making a small incision in the lower back, directly above the affected disc.

Muscle Displacement: Surrounding muscles and tissues are gently moved aside to expose the spine, allowing clear access to the herniated disc.

Disc Localization: Using imaging guidance, such as fluoroscopy, the surgeon identifies the exact location of the herniated disc and the nerves affected.

Disc Removal: The herniated portion of the disc is carefully removed using surgical tools to relieve pressure on the spinal nerves.

Closure: Once the disc material is removed, the surgeon closes the incision with sutures or staples, ensuring the wound is sealed.

Anesthesia And Pain Management

Anesthesia plays a crucial role in ensuring patient comfort and safety during lumbar discectomy. General anesthesia is commonly administered, which means the patient remains unconscious throughout the surgery. This not only prevents pain but also allows the surgical team to work without interruption.

Post-surgery, pain management is tailored to each patient's needs. Pain relievers are administered either through intravenous (IV) medications or oral pills to control discomfort as the anesthesia wears off. The medical team monitors pain levels closely to adjust medication and ensure the patient's comfort during the recovery process.

Duration And Expectations

Lumbar discectomy typically lasts between 1 to 2 hours, depending on the complexity of the herniation and the surgical approach. Patients can generally expect to stay in the hospital for a day or two for observation and initial recovery. During this time, medical staff monitor vital signs, manage pain, and ensure there are no immediate post-surgical complications.

In terms of recovery expectations, patients often experience relief from leg pain caused by nerve compression almost immediately after surgery. However, full recovery varies from person to person and may involve physical therapy to strengthen the back muscles and prevent future issues.

Role of the Surgical Team

The Surgical Team For A Lumbar Discectomy Typically Includes:

Surgeon: Leads the operation, performing the actual discectomy and ensuring the procedure is conducted safely and effectively.

Anesthesiologist: Administers anesthesia and monitors the patient's vital signs throughout the surgery.

Nurses and Surgical Technicians: Assist the surgeon, handle instruments, and provide support to the patient before, during, and after surgery.

Each member of the team plays a vital role in ensuring the procedure is successful and the patient receives optimal care.

Immediate Post-surgical Care

Immediately after lumbar discectomy, patients are closely monitored in a recovery area to ensure they wake up from anesthesia safely and comfortably. Vital signs are checked regularly, and pain management continues as needed to keep the patient comfortable.

Patients may be encouraged to start moving as soon as possible to prevent stiffness and promote circulation.

Depending on the surgical approach and the patient's condition, some individuals may be able to go home the same day, while others may require an overnight stay for observation.

Before discharge, patients receive instructions on wound care, pain management, and activity restrictions. Follow-up appointments are scheduled to monitor recovery progress and address any concerns that may arise.

CHAPTER SIX

POSTOPERATIVE RECOVERY

After undergoing a lumbar discectomy, understanding the nuances of postoperative recovery is crucial for a smooth healing process. This section breaks down the essential aspects of recovery, ensuring you are well-prepared for each step.

Hospital Stay And Initial Recovery Period

Immediately following the surgery, patients are typically monitored in the hospital for a short period. The duration of your hospital stay can vary but usually lasts from a few hours to a couple of days, depending on the complexity of the surgery and your overall health.

During this initial recovery period, nurses and medical staff will closely observe your vital signs, such as heart rate, blood pressure, and respiratory function. It's common to feel groggy or disoriented from the anesthesia, but these effects usually wear off within a few hours. You may also experience some discomfort or pain at the surgical site, which is a normal part of the healing process.

The medical team will also assess your ability to move, stand, and walk a short distance. Early mobilization is encouraged to reduce the risk of complications such as blood clots. Before being discharged, you will receive detailed instructions on wound care, activity restrictions, and signs of potential complications to watch for.

Pain Management And Medications

Effective pain management is a critical component of the postoperative recovery process. Your healthcare provider will prescribe a combination of medications to manage pain and reduce inflammation. These may include:

Analgesics: Medications like acetaminophen to alleviate mild to moderate pain.

Nonsteroidal Anti-Inflammatory Drugs (NSAIDs): These help reduce inflammation and pain.

Opioids: For severe pain, opioids may be prescribed for a short period. It is important to use these medications strictly as directed to avoid dependency.

In addition to medications, other pain management strategies such as applying ice packs to the surgical area and using a lumbar support cushion while sitting can provide relief. Keeping the surgical area elevated when resting can also help reduce swelling and discomfort.

Physical Therapy And Rehabilitation

Physical therapy is an essential part of the recovery process following a lumbar discectomy. Your surgeon will likely recommend starting physical therapy within a few weeks post-surgery.

The goal of physical therapy is to restore mobility, strengthen the muscles supporting the spine, and improve overall function.

A physical therapist will design a personalized rehabilitation program tailored to your specific needs. Initial sessions may focus on gentle stretching and low-impact exercises to enhance flexibility and reduce stiffness. As your recovery progresses, you will gradually incorporate strengthening exercises to rebuild muscle strength and support your spine.

Regular physical therapy sessions, combined with a home exercise program, can significantly enhance your recovery and prevent future back problems. Consistency and adherence to the prescribed exercises are key to achieving the best outcomes.

Activities To Avoid During Recovery

During the recovery period, it is crucial to avoid certain activities that could hinder the healing process or exacerbate your condition. Some activities to avoid include:

Heavy lifting: Avoid lifting objects heavier than 5-10 pounds to prevent strain on the spine.

Bending and twisting: Refrain from excessive bending or twisting motions, especially in the first few weeks post-surgery.

High-impact activities: Activities such as running, jumping, or contact sports should be avoided until you receive clearance from your healthcare provider.

Prolonged sitting or standing: Avoid sitting or standing for extended periods. If you need to sit, use a chair with good lumbar support and take frequent breaks to move around.

Adhering to these restrictions is crucial for a smooth and successful recovery. Gradually, as your spine heals and strengthens, your healthcare provider will guide you on when and how to reintroduce these activities safely.

Signs Of Complications And When To Seek Help

While complications from lumbar discectomy are relatively rare, it is important to be vigilant and recognize the signs that may indicate a problem. Contact your healthcare provider immediately if you experience any of the following symptoms:

Severe or worsening pain: Intense pain that is not relieved by prescribed medications.

Fever Or Chills: A Sign Of Possible Infection.

Redness, swelling, or drainage at the incision site: Indicators of infection or poor wound healing.

Numbness or weakness: Persistent numbness or weakness in the legs or feet, which could indicate nerve damage.

Difficulty urinating or loss of bowel control: These symptoms require urgent medical attention as they may signal a serious complication.

Being proactive about your recovery and aware of potential complications can significantly improve your overall outcome. Regular follow-up appointments with your surgeon are essential to monitor your progress and address any concerns promptly.

CHAPTER SEVEN

LONG-TERM CARE AND OUTCOMES

Long-term care following lumbar discectomy is crucial for ensuring a successful recovery and minimizing the risk of recurrence or complications. The primary focus is on restoring function, reducing pain, and enhancing the overall quality of life. This involves a multidisciplinary approach, incorporating medical follow-ups, physical therapy, and lifestyle changes.

Patients will typically have scheduled visits with their healthcare provider to monitor progress and address any concerns. Imaging studies, such as MRI or X-rays, may be periodically performed to assess the healing process and ensure that no new issues have arisen. Pain management strategies, including medications or nerve blocks, might be employed to help patients cope with residual pain.

Adherence to prescribed physical therapy and exercise regimens is emphasized during these follow-ups.

Consistent communication with healthcare providers allows for adjustments in the recovery plan, tailored to the patient's evolving needs and condition. Education on proper body mechanics, posture, and ergonomics is often provided to help patients protect their spine and prevent future injuries.

Long-Term Physical Therapy

Long-term physical therapy is a cornerstone of the rehabilitation process after lumbar discectomy. The goal is to restore mobility, strength, and flexibility while preventing further injury. Physical therapists work closely with patients to design individualized exercise programs that progress through different stages of recovery.

Initially, therapy focuses on gentle movements and exercises to reduce pain and inflammation. As healing progresses, the intensity and complexity of exercises are gradually increased. Core strengthening exercises are particularly important as they help stabilize the spine and support overall function. Stretching routines aim to improve flexibility and reduce muscle tightness around the affected area.

Education on proper techniques for lifting, bending, and sitting is provided to minimize strain on the spine. Physical therapists also teach patients how to incorporate these exercises into their daily routines, ensuring long-term adherence and benefits. Regular evaluations and adjustments to the exercise plan help address any challenges and ensure continuous improvement.

Maintaining Spine Health

Maintaining spine health post-surgery is vital to prevent recurrence and ensure long-term well-being. Patients are encouraged to adopt habits and practices that promote a healthy spine, which involves a combination of physical activity, ergonomic adjustments, and self-care routines.

Engaging in regular low-impact exercises such as walking, swimming, or cycling helps maintain spinal flexibility and strength. Core-strengthening exercises should be continued as they play a crucial role in supporting the spine. Patients are advised to avoid high-impact activities that could strain the back.

Ergonomic adjustments in daily life are essential. This includes using supportive chairs, maintaining proper posture, and ensuring that workspaces are designed to minimize strain. Patients should be mindful of their posture when sitting, standing, or sleeping, using cushions or supports as needed to maintain alignment.

Maintaining a healthy weight is also important as excess weight can put additional strain on the spine. A balanced diet rich in anti-inflammatory foods and adequate hydration supports overall health and healing. Patients should also avoid smoking, as it can impede healing and increase the risk of complications.

Lifestyle Adjustments For Better Outcomes

Making lifestyle adjustments can significantly improve outcomes after lumbar discectomy. Patients are encouraged to embrace changes that support their recovery and overall spine health. This involves modifying activities, incorporating healthy habits, and managing stress effectively.

One key adjustment is learning to pace activities to avoid overexertion. Patients should listen to their bodies and take breaks when needed, gradually increasing their activity levels as they build strength and endurance. This balanced approach helps prevent setbacks and promotes steady progress.

Incorporating regular exercise into daily life is crucial. Patients should aim for a mix of cardiovascular, strength, and flexibility exercises. Joining a group class or working with a personal trainer familiar with post-surgical recovery can provide additional motivation and guidance.

Stress management is also important, as stress can exacerbate pain and hinder recovery. Practices such as mindfulness, meditation, or yoga can help manage stress levels. Ensuring adequate sleep and using proper sleep hygiene practices support both physical and mental health.

Potential Long-Term Complications

While most patients experience significant improvement after lumbar discectomy, there are potential long-term complications that should be monitored.

These complications can include recurrent disc herniation, chronic pain, or the development of scar tissue around the surgical site.

Recurrent disc herniation is a possibility and may occur if the underlying issues that caused the initial herniation are not addressed.

Patients should be vigilant about maintaining spine health and following their rehabilitation program to minimize this risk.

Chronic pain can sometimes persist even after surgery. This may be due to nerve damage, inflammation, or other factors. Effective pain management strategies, including medications, physical therapy, or alternative therapies like acupuncture, can help manage chronic pain.

Scar tissue formation, known as epidural fibrosis, can also cause pain or nerve compression. If significant, this may require further medical intervention.

 Regular follow-ups with healthcare providers help detect and address these issues early, ensuring timely treatment and better outcomes.

Success Rates And Patient Stories

The success rates for lumbar discectomy are generally high, with many patients experiencing significant relief from pain and improved function.

Studies show that a large percentage of patients return to their normal activities and enjoy a better quality of life post-surgery.

Patient stories often highlight the positive impact of lumbar discectomy on their lives. Many report a drastic reduction in pain, increased mobility, and the ability to return to activities they enjoy. These stories provide hope and motivation for those considering the surgery, illustrating the potential for a successful outcome.

For instance, a patient who was unable to work or engage in hobbies due to severe pain may describe their journey through surgery and rehabilitation.

They might share how physical therapy helped them regain strength and confidence, ultimately allowing them to resume their career and enjoy time with their family. Such testimonials underscore the benefits of the procedure and the importance of comprehensive post-operative care.

CHAPTER EIGHT

COMMON CONCERNS AND FAQS

Addressing Common Patient Concerns

One of the most common concerns for patients considering lumbar discectomy is the fear of surgery itself. Many worry about the risks involved, the pain they might experience, and the recovery process. It's important to understand that lumbar discectomy is a well-established procedure with a high success rate. Surgeons use advanced techniques and state-of-the-art equipment to minimize risks and improve outcomes. Patients are encouraged to discuss their fears and ask questions during consultations to alleviate anxiety.

Another major concern is the potential for recurrence of symptoms. While lumbar discectomy effectively relieves pressure on the spinal nerves, leading to significant pain relief, there's always a possibility that disc herniation could recur. Surgeons typically provide comprehensive advice on lifestyle changes and exercises to reduce this risk. Patients should follow these recommendations diligently to maintain long-term results.

Pain management is also a crucial concern. Post-operative pain is a normal part of the healing process, but it can be managed effectively with medication and physical therapy. Patients should communicate openly with their healthcare team about their pain levels and follow prescribed pain management protocols to ensure a comfortable recovery.

Detailed FAQ Section

What is lumbar discectomy? Lumbar discectomy is a surgical procedure designed to remove a portion of a herniated disc in the lower back. This relieves pressure on the spinal nerves, reducing pain, numbness, and weakness in the legs.

Who is a candidate for lumbar discectomy? Candidates typically include individuals with herniated discs who have not responded to conservative treatments such as physical therapy, medications, or epidural injections. Severe pain, neurological deficits, or significant impairments in daily activities often indicate the need for surgery.

What can I expect during the surgery? The surgery is usually performed under general anesthesia. A small incision is made in the lower back, and the surgeon removes the portion of the herniated disc compressing the nerve. The procedure typically takes about one to two hours.

How long is the recovery period? Recovery times vary, but most patients can return to light activities within a few weeks. Full recovery, including the resumption of more strenuous activities, may take several months. Adhering to post-operative care instructions is crucial for a smooth recovery.

Are there risks involved with lumbar discectomy? As with any surgery, there are risks, including infection, bleeding, nerve damage, and recurrence of disc herniation. However, these risks are relatively low, and the procedure has a high success rate in relieving symptoms.

Tips For A Smooth Recovery

Recovery from lumbar discectomy involves several key steps to ensure the best possible outcome. First, it's essential to follow all post-operative instructions provided by your surgeon. These may include guidelines on wound care, activity restrictions, and medication schedules.

Pain management is a critical aspect of recovery. Take prescribed pain medications as directed and report any severe or persistent pain to your healthcare provider. Ice packs can also help reduce swelling and discomfort in the surgical area.

Physical therapy often plays a significant role in recovery.

A physical therapist can design a personalized exercise program to strengthen the muscles around your spine, improve flexibility, and prevent future injuries. Engaging in these exercises regularly is vital for regaining full function.

Proper nutrition and hydration support the healing process. A balanced diet rich in vitamins and minerals can accelerate recovery and boost your immune system. Staying hydrated helps maintain overall health and aids in tissue repair.

Finally, avoid heavy lifting and strenuous activities until cleared by your surgeon. Gradually increase your activity level as you heal, and listen to your body to avoid overexertion.

Managing Expectations Post-Surgery

Setting realistic expectations is crucial for a successful recovery. While lumbar discectomy can significantly reduce or eliminate pain caused by a herniated disc, it may not eliminate all symptoms immediately. Some patients experience residual numbness or weakness, which typically improves over time.

Understand that recovery is a gradual process. Initial improvements may be followed by periods of slower progress, and occasional setbacks are normal. Patience and persistence are key during this time.

It's also important to recognize the role of lifestyle changes in maintaining long-term results. Engaging in regular physical activity, maintaining a healthy weight, and practicing good posture can help prevent future disc problems. Your healthcare provider can offer specific advice tailored to your needs.

Resources For Further Information And Support

For those seeking additional information and support, several resources are available. Reputable websites such as the American Academy of Orthopaedic Surgeons (AAOS) and the North American Spine Society (NASS) offer comprehensive information on lumbar discectomy and spine health.

Support groups and online forums can provide valuable insights and emotional support from others who have undergone similar procedures. Connecting with these communities can help you feel less isolated and more empowered during your recovery journey.

Your healthcare team is also a valuable resource. Don't hesitate to reach out with any questions or concerns you may have. Regular follow-up appointments are essential for monitoring your progress and addressing any issues that arise.

By staying informed and proactive, you can navigate the recovery process with confidence and achieve the best possible outcome from your lumbar discectomy.

www.ingramcontent.com/pod-product-compliance
Lightning Source LLC
Chambersburg PA
CBHW071842210526
45479CB00001B/252